I0472554

AYURVEDIC HOME REMEDIES

BY: NIRAJ SHARMA

Ayurveda or Ayurvedic medicine is the traditional holistic medical system in India. Natural scientists and Ancient seers developed this system based on centuries of experiments, studies, and meditations.

Indian Ayurveda is a well-known system of Hindu traditional medicine of Vedic tradition, and a form of the alternative medicine. Some of the most renowned Ayurvedic texts include the Charaka Saṃhitā and Suśrutha Saṃhita. These Sanskrit texts are among the foundational compiled works of Ayurveda that helps know the history of Ayurveda.

Features of Ayurveda

Ayurveda is a science that considers the patient as a whole and provides the unequaled methods of making him/ her perfectly healthy. Apart from nature, survival of humans will become impossible within a few decades from now. Here we have listed out the common features of Ayurveda.

- It is an herbal and natural health care system
- Ayurvedic products are completely safe

Author: NIRAJ SHARMA

- Mind, body and spirit health care system for long creative life

- Treats the whole person and subtly eliminates the cause of the disease

- It gives emphasis in preventive medicine

- It is the most effective natural treatment to detoxify the body

How Does Ayurvedic Medicine Work?

Ayurvedic practitioners use a well-balanced healthy diet, lifestyle changes, stress relief and various herbal remedies to heal all sorts of conditions by helping to bring the body back into balance. The overall belief is that disease and suffering results from an imbalance in the three *doshas*, which are ways of categorizing the body's three basic energy types: Vata, Pitta and Kapha.

According to Ayurvedic medicine, everyone is unique in terms of his or her individual balance between these three energy (or personality) types. Everyone has some vata, pitta and kapha to their personality, but usually one or two of the doshas are more dominant in a particular person — and this ultimately governs body type, appetite, energy levels, moods and tendencies. Each dosha has both physical and emotional characteristics, so Ayurvedic practitioners use the three doshas to describe common traits of someone's body type and personality.

Unlike the one-size-fits-all approach to western medical treatment that fails to address the huge diversity among patients, Ayurveda takes into account individuality when prescribing holistic treatments.

As the Center for Rheumatic Diseases located in Prune, India, described it, "Every creation inclusive of a human being is a model of the universe. In this model, the basic matter and the dynamic forces (Dosha) of the nature determine health and disease, and the medicinal value of any substance (plant and mineral). The Ayurvedic practices (chiefly that of diet, lifestyle and the Panchkarama) aim to maintain the Dosha equilibrium...therapy is customized to the individual's constitution (known as Prakruti)."

Author: NIRAJ SHARMA

CONTENTS

Author: NIRAJ SHARMA

DEDICATION

This Book Is Dedicated To my Grandmom and my neighbor Mr. Acharya ji(Ayurved consultant) Who Helped Me To Write This Books On Ayurveda. Ayurveda is the ancient theory which helps to treat a health problem by simple home made things.

Author: NIRAJ SHARMA

1 .Acne

REMEDIES FOR ACNE

1. Acne affects 60% of youngsters between 12 to 24 years of age
2. It causes embarrassment, depression and lack of confidence

CAUSES

- The body is unable to remove toxins through excretion leading to contamination of the bloodstream.
- This can be due to
1. Constipation
2. Irregular bowel movement
3. Irregular meal timings

Excess starch, sugar, oil and fat consumption

SYMPTOMS

- Whiteheads

- Blackheads

- Pimples

- Red and itchy rashes

1.Natural home remedy using garlic

- Take 2-3 garlic cloves Crush them to make a paste

- Apply this paste on the affected parts

of the skin

- For sensitive skin, mix yogurt in the garlic paste before applying

2.Natural home remedy using garlic

- Consume three cloves of garlic everyday

for 1 month

- Natural home remedy using coriander leaves and turmeric powder

3.Take a handful of washed coriander leaves

1.Crush them finely

2. Place the paste on a sieve and press to extract the juice

3.Add a pinch of turmeric powder

Author: NIRAJ SHARMA

4. Mix well

5. Apply this mixture on the face every

night

Tips

- Drink ample water

- Include lots of fruits and vegetable in your diet

- Cleanse and exfoliate your face regularly

ACNE SCARS

Popping or scratching acne can leave scars

SIMPLE TECHNIQUES

method1.

Natural home remedy using aloevera

- Take an aloe vera leaf

- Peel the outer green covering

- Extract the gel from inside

- Apply the gel 2 times a day

- Leave it for 30 minutes

- Wash it off

Author: NIRAJ SHARMA

Method 2

- Natural home remedy using honey, lemon juice, almond oil and milk
- Take 1 tbsp of honey
- Add 1 tbsp lemon juice
- Add 1 tbsp almond oil
- Add 2 tbsp of milk
- Mix Well
- Apply on the affected area

These remedies are based on the principles of Ayurveda, the ancient Indian science of healing, and are completely natural, non-invasive, and can be prepared at home. Consult your doctor if the symptoms persist. Refer to the terms of use.

Author: NIRAJ SHARMA

2. Natural Ayurvedic Home Remedies for Alcoholism

REMEDIES FOR ALCOHOLISM

- Alcoholism is a psychological condition
- Addiction to alcohol can affect one's life
- negatively
- Family support and encouragement is critical to
- help quit drinking

SYMPTOMS

- Depression
- Anxiety
- Irritability
- Regular absence from work
- Insomnia
- Frequent intoxicated state

SIMPLE TECHNIQUES

method1. Natural home remedy using carom seeds

- Take 500 g of carom seeds

Author: NIRAJ SHARMA

- Add them to 8 L of water
- Boil the mixture till about 2 L water is left
- Filter the mixture
- Drink 3-4 tbsp whenever you get a
- craving for alcohol

METHOD 2.

Natural home remedy using apple juice

- Drink 2 glasses of apple juice everyday to reduce the craving

These remedies are based on the principles of Ayurveda, the ancient Indian science of healing, and are completely natural, non-invasive, and can be prepared at home. Consult your doctor if the symptoms persist. Refer to the terms of use.

Author: NIRAJ SHARMA

3. Allergies -
Natural Home Remedies for Allergies

REMEDIES FOR ALLERGIES

- An allergic reaction occurs when the immune system reacts abnormally to certain stimuli
- Reactions to allergens vary from child to child

SYMPTOMS

- Runny nose
- Chest congestion
- Sneezing
- Hives
- Rashes
- Anaphylactic attack

SIMPLE TECHNIQUES

Method1.

Natural home remedy using carrot juice,

- Beetrootnd cucumber juice
- Take 100 ml carrot juice

Author: NIRAJ SHARMA

- Add 50 ml beetroot juice
- Add 50 ml cucumber juice
- Mix well
- Give this mixture to the child once every day. This will heal the allergic reaction and prevent it from spreading.

Method2.

Natural home remedy using lemon and honey

- Take 1 glass lukewarm water
- Add 4 tbsp lemon juice
- Add 1 tsp honey
- Mix well
- Let the child drink this on an empty stomach.

Tips

- **Be observant & try to identify the allergens**
- **Most common food allergies are**
- Milk
- Eggs

Author: NIRAJ SHARMA

- Peanuts
- Soybeans
- Wheat
- Fish
- Insect bites may also trigger allergies.Get your kid diagnosed at earliest

These remedies are based on the principles of Ayurveda, the ancient Indian science of healing, and are completely natural, non-invasive, and can be prepared at home. Consult your doctor if the symptoms persist. Refer to the terms of use.

Author: NIRAJ SHARMA

4 Alzheimer's disease

REMEDIES FOR ALZHEIMER'S DISEASE

- Alzheimer's is the most common form of dementia.

- Dementia is the inability of the brain to function properly due to old age.

- It is a degenerative neurological disorder.

CAUSES

- Gradual fall in level of neurotransmitters in the brain, which are responsible for transmitting messages in the brain

- Presence of abnormal protein bundles in brain which leads to loss of connection between the brain cells

SYMPTOMS

1. Difficulty in recognizing known people or things Inability to remember recent activities or events

2. Forgetting common words while speaking, reading or writing

3. Inability to do routine chores like bathing, grooming or eating

4. Highly emotional behaviour

5. Depression and anxiety

SIMPLE TECHNIQUES

Author: NIRAJ SHARMA

Method1.

Natural home remedy using almonds

1. Soak 7-8 almonds in water overnight

2. Peel off the skin in the morning

3. Eat them on an empty stomach

4. Do this for 3-4 months

Method 2.

Natural home remedy using lemon/

peppermint oil(To fight the lethargy and depression

caused by Alzheimer's)

1. Take the juice of half a lemon or 5-10

2. drops of peppermint oil

3. Add it to a bowl of hot water

4. Inhale the fumes

Method3.

Natural home remedy using sesame oil

1. Put 3 drops of sesame oil in each nostril.

2. Do this twice a day.

3. Lukewarm sesame oil can also be.

4. applied on head and feet of the patient.

Author: NIRAJ SHARMA

5. REMEDIES FOR AMNESIA

REMEDIES FOR AMNESIA

Amnesia refers to partial or a total memory loss

Amnesia is of two types

- Anterograde
- Retrogra

CAUSES

1. Accident or brain trauma
2. Age
3. Excessive alcohol
4. Illicit drugs

SYMPTOMS

Anterograde amnesia

1. Person cannot remember any new information
2. Affects short term memory
3. Patient continuously forgets events, people, information at short intervals

Author: NIRAJ SHARMA

Retrograde amnesia

1. Patient can remember new events, but forgets the past

2. The patient forgets events or information from the period before the onset of the condition

SIMPLE TECHNIQUES

Method1.

Natural home remedy using almonds and butter

1. Soak 7-8 almonds in water overnight

2. Peel and crush them in the morning

3. Add 1 tsp of butter

4. Mix well

5. Eat this every morning

Method 2.

Natural home remedy using cumin powder and honey

1. Take 2 tsp of cumin powder

2. Add 1 tbsp honey

3. Eat every morning

Author: NIRAJ SHARMA

6. Anaemia

REMEDIES FOR ANAEMIA

1. Anaemia is a common blood disorder
2. Anaemic patients have low red blood cell count These cells are responsible for delivering oxygen from the lungs to other body parts

CAUSES

1. Iron deficiency
2. Loss of blood, especially during menstruation
3. Reduced levels of erythropoietin, a hormone produced by the kidneys

SYMPTOMS

1. Weakness
2. Dizziness
3. Fatigue
4. Lack of energy
5. Premature wrinkling
6. Droopy eyes
7. Weak memory
8. Breathlessness on exertion

Author: NIRAJ SHARMA

9. Headache

10.   Slow healing

11.   Hair loss

12.   Palpitations

Method

1. Take cold water baths 2 times every day

2. Expose yourself to the morning sun

3. Avoid tea and coffee as they hamper absorption of iron

Author: NIRAJ SHARMA

7. WEIGHT LOSS

- Being overweight is harmful to one's self esteem
- It is also a health concern since it leads to many serious ailments including:

1) Diabetes

2) High blood pressure

CAUSES

1. Some people overeat when they are:

2. Depressed

3. Bored

4. Angry

5. In a relaxed environment

a. Incorrect lifestyle

b. Improper diet

c. Lack of exercise

d. Hypothyroidism

SIMPLE TECHNIQUES

Methid1.

Natural home remedy for weight loss using black pepper powder, lemon juice and honey

Author: NIRAJ SHARMA

1. Take 1 glass lukewarm water

2. Add 1 tsp black pepper powder

3. Add 4 tbsp lemon juice

4. Add 1 tsp honey

5. Mix well

6. Drink every day

TIPS

Exercise regularly

Cabbage is very effective in burning body fat. Consume 1 bowl of cabbage everyday

Author: NIRAJ SHARMA

8. HEADACHE

Headache refers to any pain or discomfort in and around the head and neck

CAUSES

Chronic headache could be indicative of an underlying ailment

The other causes of headache include:

1. Stress
2. Lack of sleep
3. Physical exhaustion

SIMPLE TECHNIQUES

Method1.

Natural home remedy using green tea and lemon

1. Add a green tea bag
2. Squeeze ½ a lemon
3. Mix well
4. Drink for instant relief

Method2.

Natural home remedy using lemon rind

Author: NIRAJ SHARMA

1. Separate the rind (outer covering) of 2-3 lemons

2. Chop and crush the lemon rind to make a paste

3. Apply on the forehead for quick relief

   Method3.

   Natural home remedy using watermelon and sugar

1. Take 2 tbsp of cinnamon powder

2. Add water to make paste

3. Mix well

4. Apply on the temple and forehead for relief

   Tips: For chronic headaches:

1. Drink water mixed with honey every morning

2. Drink this on an empty stomach

Author: NIRAJ SHARMA

9. OSTEOARTHRITIS

OSTEOARTHRITIS

1. Arthritis affects the joints causing severe pain

2. This pain can make a person immobile

3. It is one of the most common joint disorders

   which occurs with age

CAUSES

1. Wear and tear of the cartilage, a cushion between the bones and joints

2. Increases the friction between the bones

3. Leads to stiffness and pain in the joints

4. Overweight

5. Injury

6. Excessive exercising

7. Hereditary factors

SYMPTOMS

1. Swelling and pain in the affected joint

2. Cracking noise on any joint movement

3. Constant stiffness

Author: NIRAJ SHARMA

Method1.

Natural home remedy using potato

1. Wash and cut an unpeeled potato into thin slices

2. Soak them in water overnight

3. Strain the water in the morning

4. Drink it first thing in the morning on an empty stomach

Method2.

Natural home remedy using mustard oil and camphor

1. Heat 1 cup of mustard oil

2. Add 10 g of camphor

3. Heat till camphor dissolves completely

4. Massage with the oil when

5. lukewarmThis increases the blood

   supply and reduces inflammation and stiffness

Method3.

Natural home remedy using sesame seeds

1. Take 100 ml of water

2. Soak 1 tsp of black sesame seeds in it overnight

3. Consume this mixture in the morning

Author: NIRAJ SHARMA

Method4. Natural home remedy using cinnamon powder and honey

1. Take 1 tsp of cinnamon powder

2. Add 1 tbsp of honey

3. Mix well

4. Have this on an empty stomach every morning

Author: NIRAJ SHARMA

10. ARTHRITIS

1. Arthritis refers to severe joint pain

2. It's an auto-immune disease

3. The pain in the joints can make a person immobile

CAUSES

1. Body's tissues are attacked by their own immune system

2. Common in people over 40 years of age

SYMPTOMS

- Pain and swelling in joints like:
- Fingers
- Legs
- Arms
- Wrists
- This pain is most severe in the morning

SIMPLE TECHNIQUES

Method1.Natural home remedy using mustard oil and camphor

1. Take 1 cup mustard oil

2. Add 10 g camphor

Author: NIRAJ SHARMA

3. Heat the oil till the camphor dissolves completely

4. Massage lukewarm oil on the affected area This will help improve the blood

5. Circulation in the area and will reduce the inflammation and stiffness.

Method2.

Natural home remedy using potato

1. Take a few unpeeled potato slices.

2. Soak in 1 glass cold water overnight.

3. Drink this water on an empty stomach,

   Every morning.

Method3.

Natural home remedy using green gram and garlic cloves

1. Take 3 tbsp green gram

2. Soak in 250 ml water overnight to get sprouted gram

3. Add 2 crushed garlic cloves to the sprouted gram 3.

4. Mix well

5. Consume 2 times a day You may add salt and pepper for taste.

Author: NIRAJ SHARMA

11 .REMEDIES FOR ASCITES

Ascites is the accumulation of excess fluid in the abdominal area

CAUSES

1. Cirrhosis of liver

2. Increased pressure of liver blood flow

SYMPTOMS

- Swelling of the abdomen

- As condition worsens one experiences

- Abdominal pain

- Discomfort

- Bloating

- There is an increase in pressure on the diaphragm, causing shortness of breath

SIMPLE TECHNIQUES

Method1.

Natural home remedy using bitter gourds

1. Wash and remove the skin of 3-4 bitter gourds

Author: NIRAJ SHARMA

2. De-seed it and crush the bitter gourds

3. Place the paste on a sieve and extract

4. the juice

5. Mix equal quantity of water

6. Drink 3 times a day

Method2.

Natural home remedy using fenugreek seeds

1. Soak 3 tbsp fenugreek seeds overnight in 1 cup of water

2. Strain the water in the morning

Drink on an empty stomach

Method3.

Natural home remedy using chickpeas

1. Soak 1 cup of chickpeas overnight in water

2. Consume these the next day

3. Add salt and pepper to taste

Author: NIRAJ SHARMA

12. ASTHMA

- Asthma is a condition in which the air passages in the lungs suddenly contract

- This reduces amount of air that can pass, making breathing difficult

CAUSES

- Allergic asthma is a result of body's reaction to

- allergens like

- Causes of Non allergic asthma

- Dust

- Smoke

- Drugs

- Pollution

- Fear

- Anxiety

- Stress

- Excessive consumption of processed food

- High salt intake

- Low intake of omega 3 fatty acids and anti oxidants

- Genetic factors

Author: NIRAJ SHARMA

SYMPTOMS

- Breathlessness
- Pressure in the chest
- Cough

SIMPLE TECHNIQUES

Method 1.

Natural home remedy using honey

1. Fill a saucer with honey
2. Hold it beneath the nose and inhale
3. This helps to ease the breathing

Method2.

Natural home remedy using fenugreek Seeds, ginger and honey

1. Take 2 tbsp of fenugreek seeds
2. Mix in 1 L of water
3. Let it simmer for 30 min
4. Strain the liquid
5. Crush ginger to make 2 tsp of ginger paste
6. Press the paste on a sieve and extract juice
7. Add ginger juice to the strained liquid
8. Add 1 tsp of honey
9. Mix well

Author: NIRAJ SHARMA

10.   Drink 1 glass of the mixture every morning

Method3.

Natural home remedy using Indian gooseberry powder and honey

1. Take 2 tsp of Indian gooseberry powder

2. You may de-seed and crush 1 Indian

3. gooseberry and use it in place of the powder

4. Mix 1 tsp of honey

5. Have this once every morning

Tips

1. Breathe in clean air

2. Wear a cloth mask

3. Stay away from identified allergens

4. Avoid pets which have feathers or fur

Author: NIRAJ SHARMA

13. BAD BREATH

- Bad breath can be an embarrassing condition
- It generally results from a lack of or poor oral hygiene

CAUSES

1. Bacterial activity in mouth
2. Improper oral hygiene
3. Dry mouth
4. Digestive disorders
5. Chewing tobacco
6. Consuming garlic

SYMPTOMS

1. Unpleasant odour in breath
2. Dry mouth
3. Bad taste
4. Feeling of a coating on tongue

SIMPLE TECHNIQUES

Method1.

Natural home remedy using cinnamon

1. Take 1 cup of hot water
2. Add 3 tsp of cinnamon powder

Author: NIRAJ SHARMA

3. Mix well

4. When lukewarm, use as a mouthwash

Method2.

Natural home remedy using parsley leaves Parsley leaves are rich in chlorophyll

1. and are nature's own deodorizer.

2. Chew a few parsley leaves

Tips

1. Chew 2 cardamom seeds

2. Suck on a piece of clove after each meal

3. Eat apple or guava after each meal as it clears the food particles stuck between the teeth and prevents bacterial activity

4. Brush 2 times a day

Author: NIRAJ SHARMA

14. REMEDIES FOR ALOPECIA

Alopecia is a condition in which the immune system starts attacking the hair follicles.

CAUSES

Genetics

1. Inflammation

2. Emotional stress

3. Excessive hair styling.

4. Poor nutrition

5. Certain medications

6. Chemotherapy

7. Hormonal changes during pregnancy or

8. menopause

9. Improper functioning of the thyroid gland

10.   Scalp infections

SYMPTOMS

1. Extensive hair loss

2. Bald patches

3. Thinning hair

Author: NIRAJ SHARMA

4. Permanent baldness

SIMPLE TECHNIQUES

Natural home remedy using essential oils

1. Take 50 ml of rose water in a glass bottle.

2. Add to it 50 ml of distilled water and

3. shake well to mix them both.

4. Now add to it 15 ml of apple cider vinegar.

5. Then add 5 drops of rosemary essential oil.

6. Also add 6 drops of jojoba oil.

7. Also put in 3 drops of carrot essential oil.

8. And then 3 drops of geranium essential oil.

9. Then close the bottle firmly and shake

10.   well to mix the ingredients.

Method2.

Natural home remedy using coconut and hibiscus oil

1. Crush 5 hibiscus flowers completely in a bowl.

2. Add to it ¼ cup of pure coconut oil.

3. Now mix the ingredients till they make a

4. fine paste.

5. Then apply this paste onto slightly

6. damp scalp and hair.

Author: NIRAJ SHARMA

7. Leave it on for 2 hours and then rinse off gently with cool water and a mild shampoo.

Tips

- Handle your hair gently
- Eat iron rich food
- Exercise regularly

Author: NIRAJ SHARMA

15. REMEDIES FOR BED WETTING

- Bed-wetting is a condition when a person unintentionally urinates while sleeping

- It is highly common amongst kids between the age of 3-5 years

- However, it can affect people of any age

SYMPTOMS

- Children have an immature nervous system. It

- does not alert them when their bladder is full Small bladder is unable to retain urine produced at night

- Medical conditions like

- Urinary tract infection

- Constipation

- Diabetes

- Anaemia

- Epilepsy

SIMPLE TECHNIQUES

Method1.

Natural home remedy using Indian gooseberries, turmeric powder and honey

1. Cut, de-seed and crush 2 Indian gooseberries

Author: NIRAJ SHARMA

2. Add a pinch of turmeric powder

3. Add 1 tsp honey

4. Mix well

5. Have 1 tsp of the mixture in the morning

Method2.

Natural home remedy using milk, fennel seeds and sugar

1. Take 1 glass warm milk

2. Add 1 tsp fennel seeds

3. Take 4 tbsp of sugar

4. Add 1 glass of water to this sugar

5. Heat this mixture till it becomes a thick

6. syrup

7. Add 2 tbsp of this sugar syrup to the milk

8. Mix well

9. Drink this everyday

<u>**Tips**</u>

- Eat 2-3 walnuts and about 8-10 raisins at bedtime
- For children:
- Avoid giving them liquids at bedtime
- Make it a habit to urinate before
- sleeping

Author: NIRAJ SHARMA

16. Dry Caugh

A dry cough is a cough that is accompanied with phlegm or mucous. Most dry coughs are a reaction to an environmental allergen, pollutant or toxin. The body attempts to expel the irritant from the respiratory system by coughing itout. A dry cough can also be a symptom ofan illness or a side effect of certain medications. In the absence of a serious illness or when medications are not the cause, home remedies can be used for treatment. Natural home treatments can reduce the frequency of coughing and cansoothe throat soreness and irritation.

Method1.

1. Drink water often to add moisture to your throat. You can drink other drinks besides water if you choose, as long as they are not acidic. Acidic drinks, such as orange juice, can irritate a dry throat.Step 2Run a humidifier in your home or office to add moisture to the air in your environment.

2. Run a humidifier in your home or office to add moisture to the air in your environment.

Author: NIRAJ SHARMA

17. Poison ivy

What poison ivy looks like

Each leaf has 3 small leaflets.

It grows as a shrub (low woody plant) in the far Northern and Western United States, Canada, andaround the Great Lakes.

It grows as a vine in the East, Midwest, and South of the United States.

In spring, it grows yellow-green flowers.

It may have green berries that turn off-white in early fall.

Symptoms

- You have trouble breathing or swallowing.
- The rash covers most of yourbody.
- You have many rashes or blisters.
- You experience swelling, especially if an eyelid swells shut.
- The rash develops anywhere on your face or genitals.
- Much of your skin itches, or nothing seems to ease the itch.

SIMPLE TECHNIQUES

Method 1.

Baking Soda Baths & Pastes:

Found in most kitchens, common baking soda is a great natural remedy for the itchiness associated with a poison ivy rash. To help relieve itching, place 1/2 acup of baking soda in a bath tub

Author: NIRAJ SHARMA

filled with warm water. You can also mix 3 teaspoons of baking soda with one teaspoon of water and mix until it forms a paste. Apply this paste to the infected area to relieve itching and irritation that's associated with a poison ivy rash.

Method2.

Oatmeal Paste:

Cook a small amount of oatmeal and apply it directly to the skin as a paste. Make sure to cook it very thick so that the paste will stick tothe skin. Some sources recommend putting the oatmeal on the skin while it is very warm, as the heat from the oatmeal will eventually cool, leaving the skin dry and relieved. Make sure not toapply the oatmeal when it is too hot, as this can easily burn the skin. You may also try mixing in a teaspoon of baking soda, for an extra itch-relieving effect.

Method 3.

Organic Apple Cider Vinegar:

Apply a teaspoon of organic applecider vinegar directly to the infected skin.Apple Cider Vinegarhas a toxin-pulling action that helps suck the poison out of the pores. You can also create a warm vinegar compress using a thin cotton towel. Reapply to the skin as needed.

method4.

Aloe Vera Gel:

An ancient curative remedy for the skin, aloe vera can be used directly on the infected area. You can buy a high-quality organic

Author: NIRAJ SHARMA

version at most health-food stores, or even better, buy a plant and use the gel from inner flesh ofthe leaves. External use oforganic aloe verajuicemay also help, but is not as effective as the gel.

18. Poison oak

What poison oak looks like:

1. Each leaf has 3 small leaflets.

2. It most often grows as a shrub.

3. It can grow as a vine in the Western United States.

4. It may have yellow-white berries.

Symptoms

1. Difficulty Breathing

2. Trouble swallowing

3. Eye or facial swelling

4. Rash On Your Face, Lips, Eyes, Or Genitals

5. Rash that covers more than 25 percent of your body

6. Signs of infection, such as pus or yellow fluid leaking from blisters, or blisters that have an odor

Author: NIRAJ SHARMA

7. Fever

8. Headache

9. Nausea

10.   Swollen lymph nodes

SIMPLE TECHNIQUES

Method 1.

Baking Soda Baths & Pastes:

Found in most kitchens, common baking soda is a great natural remedy for the itchiness associated with a poison oak rash. To help relieve itching, place 1/2 acup of baking soda in a bath tub filled with warm water. You can also mix 3 teaspoons of baking soda with one teaspoon of water and mix until it forms a paste. Apply this paste to the infected area to relieve itching and irritation that's associated with a poison oak rash.

Method2.

Oatmeal Paste:

Cook a small amount of oatmeal and apply it directly to the skin as a paste. Make sure to cook it very thick so that the paste will stick tothe skin. Some sources recommend putting the oatmeal on the skin while it is very warm, as the heat from the oatmeal will eventually cool, leaving the skin dry and relieved. Make sure not toapply the oatmeal when it is too hot, as this can easily burn the skin. You may also try mixing in a teaspoon of baking soda, for an extra itch-relieving effect.

Author: NIRAJ SHARMA

Method 3.

Organic Apple Cider Vinegar:

Apply a teaspoon of organic applecider vinegar directly to the infected skin.Apple Cider Vinegarhas a toxin-pulling action that helps suck the poison out of the pores. You can also create a warm vinegar compress using a thin cotton towel. Reapply to the skin as needed.

method4.

Aloe Vera Gel:

An ancient curative remedy for the skin, aloe vera can be used directly on the infected area. You can buy a high-quality organic version at most health-food stores, or even better, buy a plant and use the gel from inner flesh ofthe leaves. External use oforganic aloe verajuicemay also help, but is not as effective as the gel.

Author: NIRAJ SHARMA

19. Home Remedies for Gastritis

Causes:-

Alcohol

- Viral and bacterial infections
- Peptic ulcer disease
- Pernicious Anemia
- High intake of spicy foods

Symptoms:-

- Abdominal bloating (tenderness and swelling [distention])
- Abdominal pain (indigestion or dyspepsia), often described as burning or gnawing
- Belching (burping)
- Dark stools
- Loss of appetite
- Nausea
- Vomiting

Author: NIRAJ SHARMA

Methods:-

1. Coconut water is just apt for treating the problem of gastritis. It gives rest to thebelly and also contains loads of vitamins and minerals. When you have gastritis, consume nothing else but coconut water throughout the day.

2. Extract the juice of potatoand drink about half cup of the juice 2-3 times everyday, but it should be consumed half an hour before meals.

3. The herb marigold is considered valuable in treating gastritis. Consume1 tbsp of this herb two times in a day.

Author: NIRAJ SHARMA

20. Home Remedies for Hair Loss

Methods:-

One of the best home remedies for treating hair loss is to massage your scalp with fingers gently. It will also aid in increasing blood circulation and lend glow to your hair.

Amla oil serves as an excellent tonic for hair conditioning. To prepare amla oil, put some dry pieces of amla in coconut oil and bring to a boil. Apply this oil on the scalp and see the wonderful results.

For nourishing your hair, apply coconut milk all over your scalp and massage it into the hair roots.

Author: NIRAJ SHARMA

21. Home Remedies for Hangover Methods:-

Drink plenty of water before going to bed as well as when you wake up in the morning.

Eating some foodstuff while and after you are drinking will slow down the rate at which alcohol enters the blood, thereby reducing the hangover.

Consume vitamin C tablets, as they lead to the breakdown of alcohol content in the body.

---THE END---

I wish you all a healthy life and if there is any health problem please follow some ayurveda tips contained in my books which are really very effective and easy to apply. The best thing of ayurveda is that there is no any side effect of ayurveda. Its very useful. Any problem you have apply these tips and i bet you will get well soon.

THANKS FOR READING MY BOOKS.

PLEASE LEAVE A REVIEW.

Author: NIRAJ SHARMA

ABOUT THE AUTHOR

Niraj Sharma, born in Rajasthan (India). He is Post-Graduated from Kolhan University (Jharkhand). He is also persuing Chartered Accountancy Course from The ICAI, and is in final level.He loves to write books on various interested topics such as Cooking, Stories, Jokes etc. He also loves to write on romance fiction and science fiction and some other these types of interesting topics, in this book he write about "Ayurveda" by collecting information from many sources for the healthy and better life of the society.

Author: NIRAJ SHARMA

www.ingramcontent.com/pod-product-compliance
Lightning Source LLC
Chambersburg PA
CBHW061226180526
45170CB00003B/1174